AIR FRYER COOKBOOK FOR BEGINNERS
2021

Easy and Delicious Recipes for Beginners.
Tastier and Crispier Food for Your Family and
Guests. Reward Yourself with Healthy,
Mouthwatering Meals.
Help Your Body Lose Weight by Eating.

Violet H.Scott

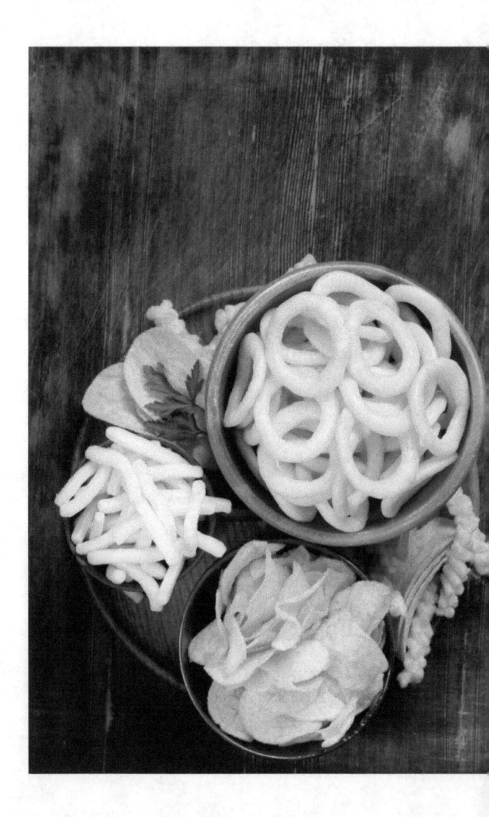

contained within this document, including, but not limited to, — errors, omissions, or inaccuracies.

Table of Contents

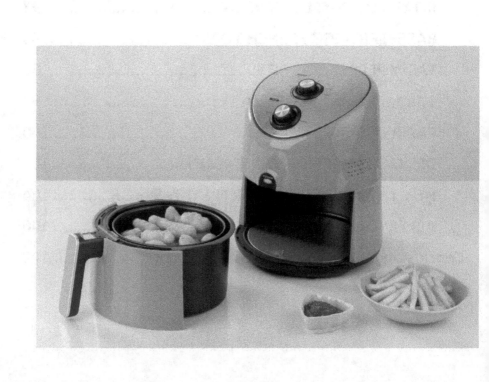

Introduction

The air fryer is a fantastic and innovative appliance,

that makes it quick and easy for you to cook delicious, healthy meals.

The air fryer does all the work. It has a thermostat that comes with overheating protection, so there will be no danger of burning your food. There's also a food weight indicator so you know the exact amount you're preparing, and a timer with an automatic shut-off feature, so you can plan your preparation as best as possible.

Non-stick, easy to clean and easy to store, practicality is one of its strengths.

In a short period of time, the air fryer will

prepare your meal, whether it's chicken, steak, fish or vegetables, frying them perfectly.

Now you can easily bake even cakes or pies, you will experience tasty desserts never eaten before.

Its great advantage is the fact that it keeps the nutritional content intact compared to cooking with a classic fryer. High cooking temperatures deprive the food of much of what our body needs.

The difference is that when food is prepared in an air fryer, it is only cooked to the safe temperatures appropriate for your health and food. It prepares healthy meals with less time, more control and healthier results. It is the most efficient way to cook.

Hot air replaces oil, creating a crisp, delicious crust.

It will cook evenly, thanks to the perfect heat distribution aided by the fan.

The calories of typical fried foods will be a distant memory, with the absence or minimal amount of oil added, will be reduced dramatically, without going to the expense of crispiness.

Your food will taste just like fried food, without coming from the oil.

Your advantages with a hot air fryer

- tasty and healthy food
- vitamin-rich food
- low-fat preparation of food
- natural taste is retained
- quick and easy cleaning thanks to the easy-care production method
- Can be used in many ways: baking, roasting, grilling, cooking, defrosting, deep-frying
- no grease odor in the house, no grease stains

- easily usable for diabetics and dieters
- Food does not lose moisture
- ideal for private individuals and (large) families
- safe and easy application
- Fry French fries with 80 percent less fat
- Food rotates in a stream of hot air and does not swim in hot fat
- Preparation of fish, meat and vegetables

A few numbers about air fryers

The body derives numerous benefits from the use of this product.

The preparation of fries requires 80 percent less fat than a regular fryer.

French fries made from fresh potatoes contain about three percent fat, those from conventional fryers up to 20 percent. Frozen fries cooked with hot air, on the other hand, have only about six percent fat. A serving of conventional fries (about 250 grams) has just under 700 calories, while hot air fries have only 500. That's why its use is becoming increasingly popular.

Keto Airfryer Recipes

AIR FRYER BUTTER ZUCCHINI VEGETABLES

30 to 60 min

185 kcal

light

Portion size For 4 people

Ingredients

600 g yellow zucchini

onion

2 Garlic cloves

1 Dossier spoon of olive oil

salt

pepper

70 g butter

Instructions

Wash and clean the zucchini and cut into bite-sized pieces of approx. 2 × 2 cm. Peel the onion and garlic, cut the onion into wedges, finely dice the garlic. Place in a bowl with the zucchini and mix with the oil. Salt and pepper.

Put the prepared ingredients in the cooking container with the paddle in place, add the butter and set the timer for 20 minutes. Start the device. If the vegetables are still too firm, simply extend the cooking time by a few minutes.

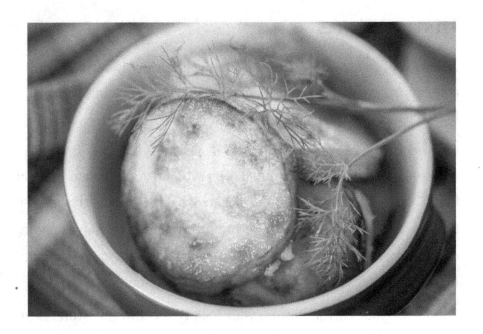

HEALTHY CARROT FRIES

Ingredients

3 carrots

3 tablespoons of olive oil

2 tablespoons of liquid honey

some salt and pepper

some thyme

Instructions

Heats the oven for your carrot fries: in the electric stove: 175 ° C / with convection: 150 ° C / with gas: level 2. Lay out a baking sheet with baking paper and then let the tube glow properly.

For your crispy carrot fries, mix the oil and honey together first. Then grab your carrots for the carrot fries, peel them, and then cut them in half. Then you cut them into thick strips so that the carrot fries get the typical fries' shape. Now divide them into thirds or halves again, depending on how big you like your fries. Mix the honey mixture into the carrot fries and let it steep for about 15 minutes.

Then bake your carrot fries on your baking sheet in the oven for 30 minutes until they are nice and crispy. Then simply take them out of the tube and put them in a large bowl like normal fries. Then season them with salt and pepper. Of course, you can also use more spices such as oregano, thyme or rosemary. Simply season them to your taste and then nibble them away with relish.

Our tip: the carrot fries are perfect for a bowl full of finger food. You can do this with Mozzarella sticks, normal fries or Vegetable chips complete. There is a snack for every taste

FAST TURKEY BURGERS RECIPE

Yield: 4

Prep time: 7 minutes

 Cook time: 12 minutes

Total time: 19 minutes

Ingredients

1 lb. ground turkey

2 garlic cloves

3/4 tsp sea salt

1/2 tsp ground black pepper

1/2 tsp dried basil

1 Tbsp olive oil

Instructions

Preheat the air fryer to 360F for 5 minutes.

Combine the ground turkey, olive oil, minced garlic, sea salt, pepper, and dried basil in a bowl.

Divide the burger mix into 4 equal size balls and flatten them into patties.

Depending on which size of air fryer you have, you'll be able to make 2 or up to 4 air fryer turkey burgers at a time.

Cook the turkey burgers in the air fryer for a total of 12 minutes, flipping after 8 minutes, or until your desired degree of doneness.

If you're making burgers with cheese, add it after you flip the burgers.

Serve hot with your favorite burger toppings like bacon, lettuce, tomatoes, onion, pickles, or avocado slices.

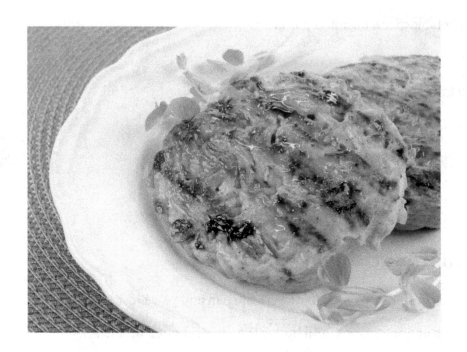

AIR FRYER CHEDDAR SCRAMBLED EGGS

Yield: 2 servings

Prep time 3 minutes

Cook time 9 minutes

Total time 12 minutes

Ingredients

1/3 tablespoon unsalted butter

2 eggs

2 tablespoons milk

salt and pepper to taste

1/8 cup cheddar cheese

Instructions

Place butter in an oven/air fryer-safe pan and place inside the air fryer.

Cook at 300 degrees until butter is melted, about 2 minutes.

Whisk together the eggs and milk, then add salt and pepper to taste.

Place eggs in pan and cook it on 300 degrees for 3 minutes, then push eggs to the inside of the pan to stir them around.

Cook for 2 more minutes then add cheddar cheese, stirring the eggs again.

Cook 2 more minutes.

Remove pan from the air fryer and enjoy them immediately.

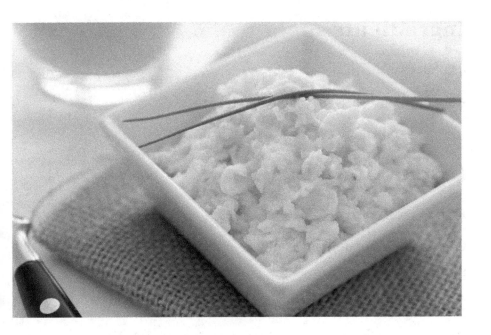

AIR FRYER SLICED HOT DOGS

Yield: 4 servings

Cook time

5 minutes

Total time

5 minutes

Ingredients

4 hot dogs

4 hot dog buns, sliced down the middle

Instructions

Preheat air fryer to 400 degrees.

Cook hot dogs for 4 minutes until cooked, moving basket once halfway through to rotate them.

Place hot dogs into hot dog buns.

Cook hot dogs in buns an additional 1-2 minutes, still at 400 degrees.

Enjoy immediately

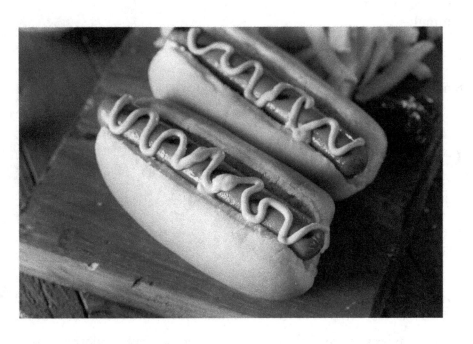

CRISPY BREAD & BACON

Yield: 4 servings

Cook time

8 minutes

Total time

8 minutes

Ingredients

7 ounces of bacon (approximately 8 slices)

1-2 pieces of bread

Instructions

Place 1-2 pieces of bread at the bottom of your air fryer underneath the basket. *

Put bacon in air fryer evenly in one layer. Cut bacon in half if too long.

Cook in air fryer at 350 degrees for 8-10 minutes, until it's at your desired crispiness. **

Enjoy immediately.

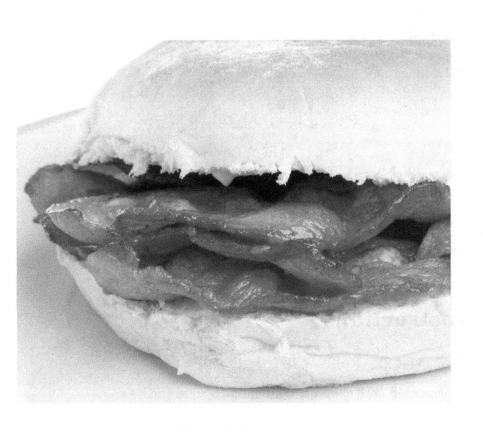

FAST AIR FRYER PORK CHOPS

Yield: 4 servings

Prep time

1 minute

Cook time

10 minutes

Total time

11 minutes

Ingredients

4 pork chops (boneless, bone-in, thin, or thick)

salt and pepper to taste

Instructions

Preheat air fryer to 400 degrees.

Season each pork chop with salt and pepper generously.

Place pork chops in the air fryer in a single layer.

Cook for 10-15 minutes*, flipping halfway through until the pork chops JUST hit 145 degrees at its thickest point.

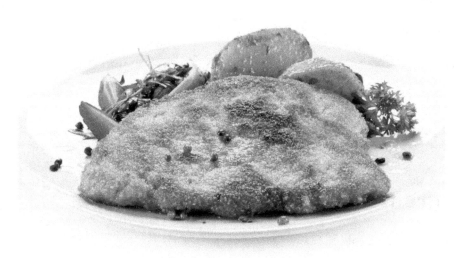

HEALTHY ROASTED CARROTS

YIELD: 4 SERVINGS

Prep time

5 minutes

Cook time

15 minutes

Total time

20 minutes

Ingredients

16 ounces of carrots

1 teaspoon oil

salt and pepper (to taste)

Instructions

Peel carrots and cut into 2-inch chunks. Cut any larger pieces in half to make all pieces a similar size.

Preheat air fryer to 360 degrees.

Toss carrots in about 1 teaspoon of oil. *

Place carrots in air fryer and cook for 15-18 minutes, shaking every few minutes.

Test carrots with a fork for tenderness. They are done when it glides through the carrot easily.

Add salt and pepper to taste and shake basket to coat.

Serve and enjoy immediate

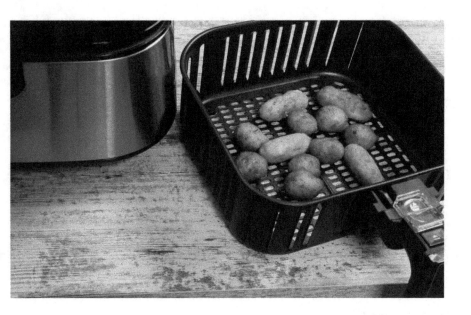

HEALTHY AIR FRYER BUFFALO CAULIFLOWER

Yield: 4 servings

Prep time

5 minutes

Cook time

11 minutes

Total time

16 minutes

Ingredients

1 head of cauliflower, cut into florets

1/4 cup buffalo sauce

Instructions

Preheat air fryer to 400 degrees.

Add cauliflower into the air fryer and cook for 7-8 minutes.

Remove cauliflower from the air fryer and place inside a bowl.

Add buffalo sauce to cauliflower and mix to coat cauliflower evenly.

Add the cauliflower back to the air fryer, turn temperature to 350 degrees, and cook for about 3 minutes.

Remove buffalo cauliflower from the air fryer and enjoy immediately.

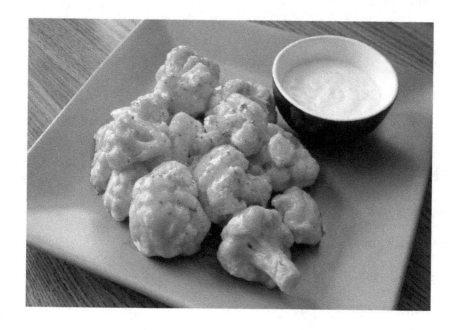

AIR FRYER BEEF HAMBURGERS

Yield: 4 hamburgers

Prep time

5 minutes

Cook time

8 minutes

Total time

13 minutes

Ingredients

1-pound ground beef, thawed (preferably 80/20)

1 clove garlic, minced

1/2 teaspoon salt

1/4 teaspoon pepper

Instructions

Preheat air fryer to 360 degrees.

Mix together the ground beef, minced garlic, salt, and pepper with your hands.

Form ground beef into 4 patties and press them down with the back of a pie plate to make them evenly flat.

Place hamburgers in a single layer inside the air fryer.

Cook for 8-12 minutes, flipping halfway through cooking for medium-well hamburgers. *

Carefully remove hamburgers from the air fryer, ** place onto hamburger buns (if using), and add desired toppings.

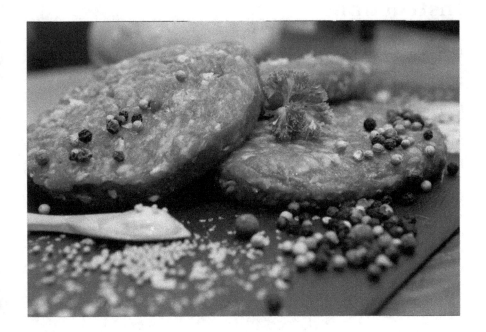

SALT & PEPPER BOILED EGGS

Yield: 4 servings

Ingredients

4 eggs

salt and pepper to taste

Instructions

Preheat air fryer to 270 degrees.

Place eggs in the air fryer, preferably on a wire rack, and cook for 15-17 minutes.

Immediately place eggs in a bowl full of cold water and ice until cool, at least 5 minutes.

Peel eggs and top with salt and pepper or refrigerate up to one week.

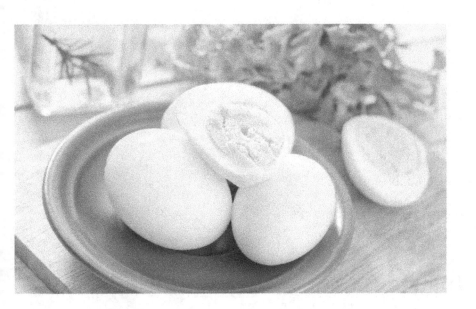

HAM & EGG CUPS (

Servings6 servings

Calories97kcal

Ingredients

6 slices prosciutto

6 eggs

1/2 cup baby spinach

1/4 tsp pepper, salt optional

Instructions

Air Fryer Egg Cups

Preheat your Air Fryer or Oven to 375.

While it preheats, lay one piece of prosciutto inside each cup, pressing to line the bottom and sides of each cup.

As long as your muffin tin is on the newer side, you do not need to spray the tin first – as the prosciutto cooks, it will naturally pull away from the tin as it cooks. If you're not sure, go ahead and spray or drizzle a little oil inside first.

Gently press about 4-5 spinach leaves into the bottom of each cup.

Crack one egg into each cup. Then just sprinkle with a little pepper and they're ready to go into the oven or air fryer.

Bake in the Air Fryer. Carefully transfer your muffin tin or muffin cups to the air fryer (leave a little space between them), and close. Cook for 10 minutes.

Bake in Oven: If using silicone muffin cups, set them on a baking sheet. Set the muffin tin or baking sheet on the middle rack and cook for 12-13 minutes for a medium-runny egg.

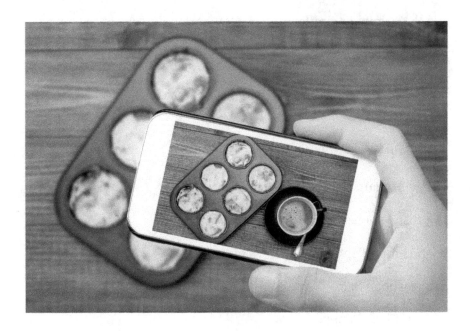

HEALTHY STEAK & CHICKEN KABOBS

Yield: 6 Servings prep time: 30 minutes cook time: 10 minutes total time: 40 minutes

Ingredients

2 Boneless Skinless Chicken Breasts

1/2 lb. Sirloin, or similar

1 Small Zucchini

1 Small Onion

1 Yellow Pepper

1 Green Pepper

Grape Tomatoes

2-3 tbsp Worcestershire Sauce

1 tsp Lemon Pepper

1/2 teaspoon Salt

1/4 tsp Black Pepper

8" Metal or Wood Skewers (Or however long your air fryer will hold.)

Instructions

Allow wooden skewers to soak for 10 minutes prior to cooking. Metal skewers do not need to soak. Rinse and slice all vegetables into 2" pieces.

Cut beef and chicken into 2" pieces. Add beef to a bowl and marinade with Worcestershire sauce, 1/2 teaspoon salt, and 1/4 teaspoon black pepper. Add chicken to a separate bowl and sprinkle with 1 teaspoon of lemon pepper.

Beginning with meat on each one, add beef and vegetables to skewers. Add chicken and vegetables to other skewers. Vegetables can be added in any order you like. Avoid adding steak and chicken to the same kabob due to different cook times.

Place kabobs in the air fryer basket in a single layer. Mine held 3 kabobs at a time. Cook in the air fryer at 400 degrees Fahrenheit for 9-10 minutes for chicken kabobs and 10-12 minutes for beef kabobs.

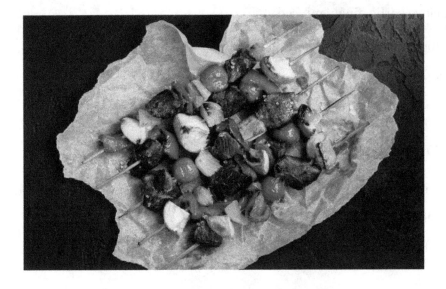

AIR FRYER TASTY SHISHITO PEPPERS

Prep Time: 5 minutes Cook Time: 4 minutes Total Time: 9 minutes
Servings: 4

Ingredients

½ lb. shishito peppers

1 tsp avocado oil or other oil with a high smoke point

Lemon Aioli

½ cup vegan mayonnaise, or your favorite mayo

2 tbsp lemon juice, freshly squeezed

1 clove garlic, finely minced

1 tbsp fresh parsley, finely chopped

¼ tsp each sea salt and pepper

Instructions

Combine all ingredients for the Lemon Aioli in a small bowl. Set aside to allow flavors to blend.

Preheat the air fryer to 390°F. for 3 minutes.

Toss shishito peppers with oil, then add to the basket of the air fryer in a single layer.

Fry for 4 minutes. Push pause and check for doneness. Peppers should be slightly softened and lightly blistered. If not done, cook for another minute or two.

Remove to a serving dish, squeeze a little fresh lemon juice overall and sprinkle with sea salt. Serve with Lemon Aioli.

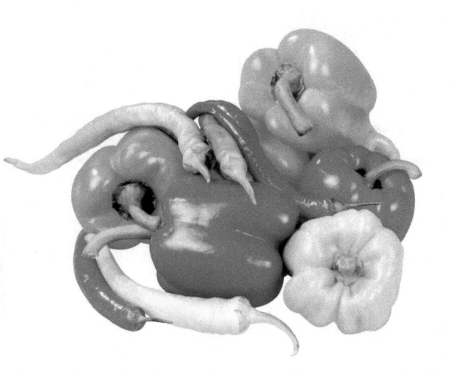

AIR FRYER BACON BRUSSELS SPROUTS

Prep Time: 5 minutes

Cook Time: 18 minutes

Total Time: 23 minutes

 Servings: 4

Ingredients

¾ to 1 lb Brussels sprouts

1 tsp olive oil

1 tsp balsamic vinegar

2 slices bacon, nitrate-free

1 pinch salt and pepper, to taste

Instructions

Wash and trim the Brussels sprouts first. Trim the tough stem end and remove any damaged leaves. Pat them dry.

Preheat your air fryer to 380°F. for 3 minutes

In a medium bowl, toss with oil and balsamic vinegar.

Cut bacon slices into one-inch pieces. Add the sprouts to the air fryer basket and top with the bacon pieces.

Air fry for 16 - 18 minutes, shaking the basket at least once partway through the cooking time.

Check for doneness with a fork and add a minute or two more frying time, if needed.

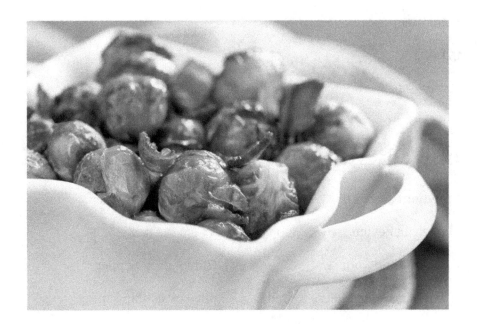

LOW CARB ZUCCHINI FRIES

Prep time

5 mins

Cook time

10 mins

Total time

15 mins

Servings 4

Ingredients

2 medium zucchinis

1 large egg beaten

⅓ cup almond flour

½ cup parmesan cheese grated

1 tsp Italian seasoning

½ tsp garlic powder

¼ tsp sea salt

¼ tsp black pepper

olive oil cooking spray

Instructions

Cut the zucchini in half and then into sticks about ½ inch thick and 3-4 inches long.

In a bowl, combine the almond flour, grated parmesan, Italian seasoning, garlic powder, sea salt, and black pepper. Mix to combine. Set aside.

In a separate bowl, whisk egg until beaten.

Dredge zucchini sticks in the egg wash and then roll and coat in the almond flour breading mixture. Place on a plate (for air fryer) or a lined baking sheet (for the oven).

Generously spray the zucchini sticks with olive oil cooking spray.

Air fryer Directions:

Working in small batches (depending on the air fryer size), place the zucchini fries in a single layer in the air fryer and air fry at 400°F (200°C) for 10 minutes or until crisp and golden.

Oven Directions:

Bake at 425°F (220°C) for 18-22 minutes, flipping them over halfway through until they are golden and crisp.

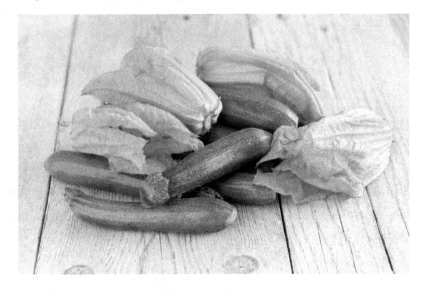

AIR FRYER RAMEKIN BAKED EGGS

Prep Time: 4 minutes

Cook Time: 16 minutes

Total Time: 20 minutes

Servings: 2

Ingredients

4 large Eggs

2 ounces Smoked gouda, chopped

Everything bagel seasoning

Salt and pepper to taste

EQUIPMENT

Air Fryer

Instructions

Spray the inside of each ramekin with cooking spray. Add 2 eggs to each ramekin, then add 1 ounce of chopped gouda to each. Salt and pepper to taste. Sprinkle your everything bagel seasoning on top of each ramekin (as much as you like).

Place each ramekin into the air fryer basket. Cook for 400F for 16 minutes, or until eggs are cooked through. Serve.

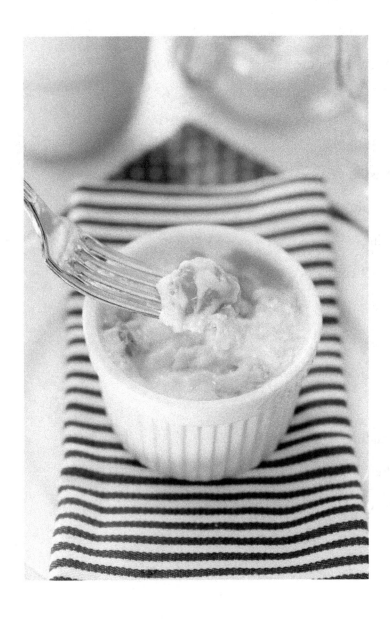

CRISPY EGGPLANT & CHEESE

Prep time 20 minutes Cook time 8 minutes Additional time

1 hour 30 minutes

Total time

1 hour 58 minutes

Ingredients

1 Medium Eggplant

Sea Salt

Filling-

6 oz. Ricotta Cheese

1/4 cup Parmesan Cheese

3 tbsp. Fresh Parsley

1 tsp Garlic Powder

1 Egg

Breading-

2 Eggs

1.5 cups Pork Rind Crumbs

2 tsp Italian Seasoning

1/4 cup Parmesan Cheese (for breading)

Instructions

Slice the eggplant into 1/2-inch rounds. Place on a paper towel lined baking sheet and sprinkle sea salt across the top. Place paper towels over that and another baking sheet. Add bowls or plates to weigh down the pan to extract excess water for 30 minutes.

While the sliced eggplant is sweating, combine the ricotta, parmesan, parsley, and one egg together in a bowl and set aside.

Remove the paper towels off of the eggplant and wipe away the excess salt. Spread a heaping tablespoon of the ricotta mixture over the top of each round and spread it evenly across the eggplant with a butter knife. Repeat with all the eggplant slices.

Place the ricotta layered eggplant rounds onto a baking sheet and place it into the freezer to set.

Once set, add the two eggs to a dish and then combine the pork rinds, 1/4 cup of parmesan, and the Italian seasonings in a separate dish. Coat each piece of eggplant in the egg wash and then in the pork rind mixture. Press down as needed to coat evenly.

Place each round back onto a baking sheet and into the freezer again to set, about 30-45 minutes.

Cooking Methods-

The Air Fryer: This is my favorite method personally and the one I suggest if you have one. Just 8 minutes at 375 F is the perfect amount of time to get a crispy golden-brown coating and perfectly cooked eggplant.

Baking: If you plan on baking, place on an elevated cooling rack to help heat the eggplant from above and underneath (no one wants soggy breading). Bake at 425 F for 12 minutes and then broil for some nice color on top if desired.

Pan Searing/Frying: Heat a frying pan to medium high heat and add a little swirl of a high smoke point oil (avocado is my go-to) and sear face down first, about 4-5 minutes per side. Use a spatula and non-stick pan to carefully flip the eggplant rounds over to finish cooking.

Serve on a plate as an appetizer or with low carb keto buns as a keto eggplant parmesan sandwich!

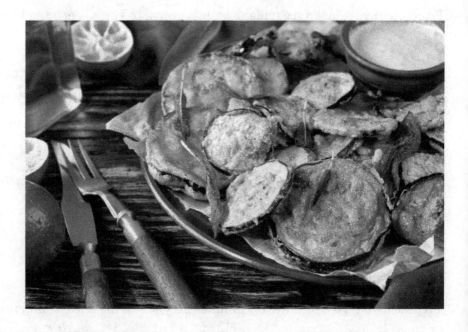

WHOLE CHICKEN WITH SPICES

Cook Time: 1-hour

Total Time: 1 hour

Yield: 1 1x

ingredients

1 3 to 4 lb. Whole Chicken

Black Pepper

Salt

Paprika

Smoked Paprika

Garlic Powder

Onion Powder

Dried Thyme

Cooking Twine (about 2-3ft.)

instructions

Place your whole chicken on a flat, clean surface and season liberally with spices, rubbing them into the skin.

Take your cooking twine and follow instructions provided in manual to truss the chicken.

Slide the rotisserie rod from the neck down, through your seasoned and trussed chicken.

Secure the rotisserie forks on each end to hold the chicken in place.

Insert the rotisserie rod into the sockets in the air fryer oven and close the door.

Turn on the oven and cycle through the oven menu to activate the rotisserie function preset. The press the actual rotisserie button and allow the cooking cycle to commence.

Once the cycle is complete, check the internal temperature of the chicken (take it out of the oven to do so with oven mitts and rotisserie tongs). If it has reached 165°F, it is down, if not, place it back in the oven and repeat the cycle process.

Place the chicken on a plate, unscrew the forks, carefully pull out the rotisserie rod, and remove the cooking twine before allowing the chicken to rest and carving as desired.

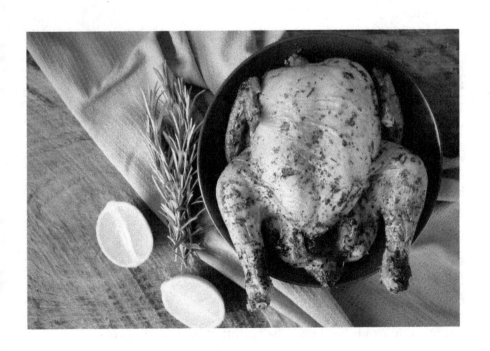

AIR FRYER BUNCH KALE

Cook time

9 minutes

Total time

9 minutes

Ingredients

1/2 bunch kale

Salt

Drizzle of olive oil

Instructions

Pre-heat the air fryer to 380.

Cut the kale from the stems, then cut that into small pieces.

Fill the bottom of a large pot about 1-inch high. Put in an expandable steamer basket.

Put the kale into the steamer basket and put the lid on the pot. Turn the heat up to high and let it steam for five minutes.

Remove the steamer basket from the pot.

Using a pair of tongs, move the kale pieces from the steamer basket to the air fryer basket.

Drizzle a tiny bit of oil (approximately 1 teaspoon or less) on the kale chips. Sprinkle them with salt.

Cook for two minutes, shake the air fryer basket, then cook for an additional two minutes.

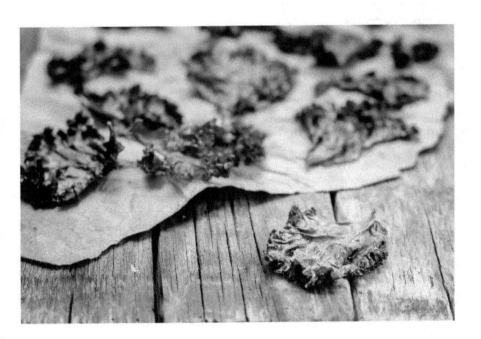

AIR FRYER RANCH JALAPENO POPPERS

Prep Time10 minutes

Cook Time10 minutes

Total Time20 minutes

Servings 4 servings

Ingredients

6 jalapenos halved and seeded

1 tbsp ranch dressing powder

4 ounces cream cheese softened

1/4 cup cheddar cheese shredded

1/4 cup green onion sliced finely

1 pound bacon

Instructions

1. Wash the jalapenos and cut them lengthwise, removing the seeds and membrane. Wear gloves if you have them

2. Combine the softened cream cheese, cheddar cheese, ranch powder, and green onions in a bowl, until well mixed.

3. Place 1-2 tbsp of filling in each jalapeno half, then wrap it in a slice of bacon.

4. Cook them in your air fryer at 400F for about 10 minutes or until the bacon is cooked and starting to crisp. Let cool and enjoy!

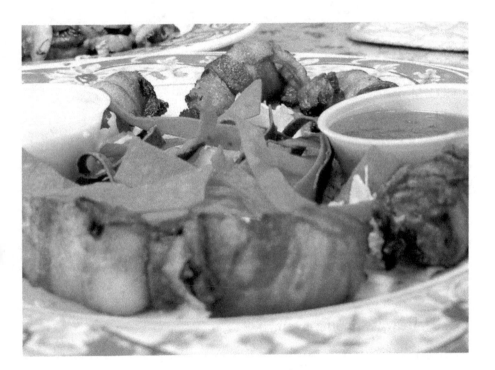

LOW CARB CHURRO STICKS!

=

Prep Time: 10 minutes

Cook Time: 8-10 minutes

Servings: 5 (4 churro sticks per serving)

Ingredients

1 ½ C. Mozzarella cheese

2 oz. Cream cheese

1 C. Almond flour

2 Tbsp. Swerve confectioners' sugar substitute

½ tsp. Cinnamon

1 ½ tsp. Baking powder

1 Egg

2 Tbsp. Heavy whipping cream

For the topping:

1 Tbsp. Butter melted

2 Tbsp. Swerve granulated sweetener

1 tsp. Cinnamon

Instructions

Preheat the air fryer to 350 degrees.

In a microwave safe bowl, combine the mozzarella cheese and cream cheese. Heat for 30 seconds at a time until the cheeses are completely melted and well blended into a dough.

Knead the almond flour, baking powder, Swerve confectioners' sugar substitute and ½ teaspoon of cinnamon into the melted cheese mixture. It is best to use your hands and be patient, as this can take a few minutes.

Blend the egg and heavy whipping cream into the dough mixture until smooth.

Spoon the dough into a piping bag or other tool with a large star shaped decorators tip on the end.

Place 3-4-inch-long strips of the dough onto a parchment lined tray.

Cook the churro sticks in the air fryer for 4-5 minutes per side or until each side is browned and the churro sticks are cooked through.

Brush the air fried churro sticks with the melted butter.

Mix together the granulated sweetener and 1 teaspoon of cinnamon in a small bowl.

Sprinkle the cinnamon over the buttered churro sticks and serve.

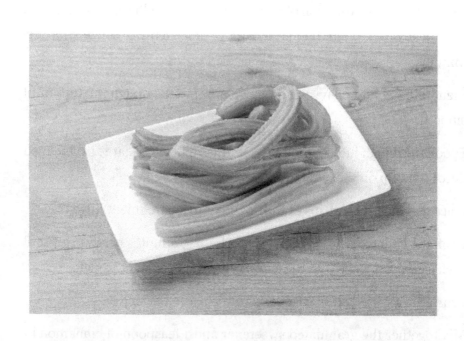

CRISPY AVOCADO FRIES

Preparation Time: 10 minutes

Cooking Time: 10 minutes

Servings: 4

Ingredients

Two avocados, peeled, pitted, and sliced

1 cup almond meal

1 tsp. salt

Directions:

Preheat your Air Fryer Oven temperature to 390 degrees F

Take a bowl and add panko breadcrumbs with salt into a bowl

Dredge the avocado fries into almond meal mixture until it properly covers

Place your avocado fries in the air fryer

Cook for 10 minutes, shake after 5 minutes

Serve and enjoy!

HEALTHY AIR FRYER TURKEY LEGS

Prep Time10 minutes

Cook Time21 minutes

Servings2

Ingredients

2 turkey legs

1 tbsp sea salt

1/2 tsp chili powder

1/2 tbsp garlic powder

1/2 tsp paprika

1/4 tsp basil

1/2 tbsp Old Bay

olive oil spray

Instructions

Preheat air fryer to 390 degrees F.

Mix together dry rub ingredients in a bowl. Rub on all sides of legs.

Spray inside of air fryer basket with olive oil spray and lay legs inside. Spray top of legs with olive oil spray.

Close drawer and cook at 390 degrees F for 21 minutes. Check at thickest part of leg to ensure internal temp. is 165 F. Remove from basket and allow to rest for 5 minutes before slicing meat off of bone and serving.

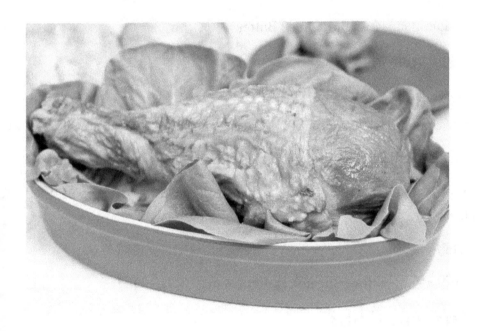

AIRYER LOW CARB SHRIMP SCAMPI

Prep Time: 5 minutes Cook Time: 10 minutes Total Time: 15 minutes

Servings: 4

Ingredients

4 tablespoons (4 tablespoons) Butter

1 tablespoon (1 tablespoon) Lemon Juice

1 tablespoon (1 tablespoon) Minced Garlic

2 teaspoons (2 teaspoons) Red Pepper Flakes

1 tablespoon (1 tablespoon) chopped chives, or 1 teaspoon dried chives

1 tablespoon (1 tablespoon) chopped fresh basil, or 1 teaspoon dried basil

2 tablespoons (2 tablespoons) Chicken Stock, (or white wine)

1 lb. (453.59 g) Raw Shrimp, (21-25 count)

Instructions

Turn your air fryer to 330F. Place a 6 x 3 metal pan in it and allow it to start heating while you gather your ingredients.

Place the butter, garlic, and red pepper flakes into the hot 6-inch pan.

Allow it to cook for 2 minutes, stirring once, until the butter has melted. Do not skip this step. This is what infuses garlic into the butter, which is what makes it all taste so good.

Open the air fryer, add butter, lemon juice, minced garlic, red pepper flakes, chives, basil, chicken stock, and shrimp to the pan in the order listed, stirring gently.

Allow shrimp to cook for 5 minutes, stirring once. At this point, the butter should be well-melted and liquid, bathing the shrimp in spiced goodness.

Mix very well, remove the 6-inch pan using silicone mitts, and let it rest for 1 minute on the counter. You're doing this so that you let the shrimp cook in the residual heat, rather than letting it accidentally overcook and get rubbery.

Stir at the end of the minute. The shrimp should be well-cooked at this point.

Sprinkle additional fresh basil leaves and enjoy.

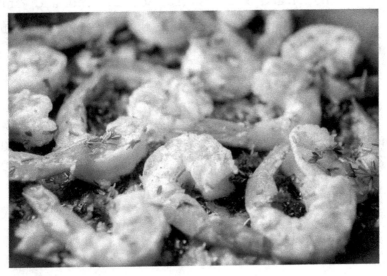

AIR FRYER CHOCOLATE COOKIES

Ingredients

½ Cup butter

⅓ Cup cream cheese

1 Egg beaten

1 Tsp vanilla extract

⅓ Cup erythritol

½ Cup coconut flour

⅓ Cup sugar-free chocolate chip cookies

Instructions

In a bowl mix butter and cream cheese. Add erythritol and vanilla extract and whip up until fluffy. Add the egg and beat until incorporated. Mix in coconut flour and chocolate chips. Let the dough rest for 10 minutes.

Scoop out around 1 Tbsp of dough and form the cookies.

Line the air fryer basket with parchment paper and place the cookies inside. Air fry for 6 minutes at 350 degrees.

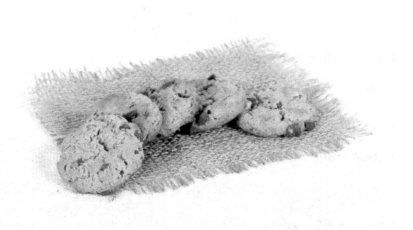

AIR FRYER SPICES CHICKEN WINGS

Prep time

10 mins

Cook time

23 mins

Marinate time

4 hrs.

Total time

4 hrs. 33 mins

Ingredients

⅓ cup extra virgin olive oil

¼ cup fresh lemon juice

2 large cloves garlic minced

2 tsp dried oregano

1 tsp fresh or ½ tsp dried thyme

2 tsp kosher salt

½ tsp coarsely ground pepper

¼ tsp crushed red pepper flakes

2 lb chicken wing drumettes

Tzatziki sauce

Instructions

Whisk together all the ingredients except the chicken and Tzaziki sauce. Put the marinade in a large resealable bag and add the chicken.

Refrigerate 4 hours to overnight, turning occasionally.

Heat air fryer to 370°F.

Add half the chicken and cook 20 minutes, turning chicken over midway.

After 20 minutes, give the air fryer basket a shake to toss the chicken a bit. Cook 2 minutes more or until juices run clear and meat is no longer pink.

Repeat with the remaining chicken. Serve with Tzatziki sauce.

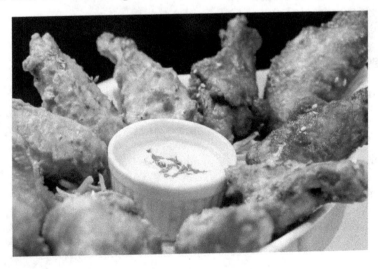

AIR FRYER KETO MUSHROOMS

Cook Time: 11 minutes

Total Time: 21 minutes Servings: 4 servings

Ingredients

2 cups Pork Rinds

1/4 cup Parmesan Cheese grated

1 Tablespoon Dried Parsley Flakes

1 teaspoon Garlic Powder

3/4 teaspoon Sea Salt

1/2 teaspoon Dried Basil

1/2 teaspoon Paprika

1 large Egg

12 ounces Cremini Mushrooms washed and patted dry

Pure Virgin Coconut Oil for greasing basket

Dipping Sauce

2 Tablespoons Butter Melted

1 clove Fresh Garlic smashed

Instructions

Carefully wash mushrooms and slice off just the bottom of the stem. Pat dry mushrooms and cut in half.

Crack an egg into a medium bowl and whisk well.

Add mushrooms to egg wash and mix to coat completely.

To the bowl of a food processor, add pork rinds, Parmesan cheese, parsley, garlic, salt, paprika and basil and process until well combined.

Dump dry mixture into a medium bowl or baggie.

Dump mushrooms with egg wash into dry mixture and shake to coat completely

Coat basket of air fryer with coconut oil and place mushrooms into basket. Lightly spray with oil.

Cook at 380 degrees for 10 minutes, shaking/turning over the mushrooms half way through.

After 10 minutes, increase temperature to 400 degrees and cook for 30 seconds to one minute to crisp. Remove mushrooms to a plate.

Serve mushrooms with garlic butter.

To Make Dipping Sauce

Smash garlic and place into microwave safe bowl. Add butter. Microwave butter for 15-20 seconds or until melted.

Instructions

Place trivet into pressure cooker and place the basket on top.

Lightly Coat basket with coconut oil and place mushrooms into basket. Lightly spray with oil.

Place it on top of Instant Pot or pressure cooker.

Cook at 375 degrees for 10 minutes, turning over the mushrooms half way through.

After 10 minutes, increase temperature to 400 degrees and cook for 30 seconds to one minute to crisp. Remove mushrooms to a plate.

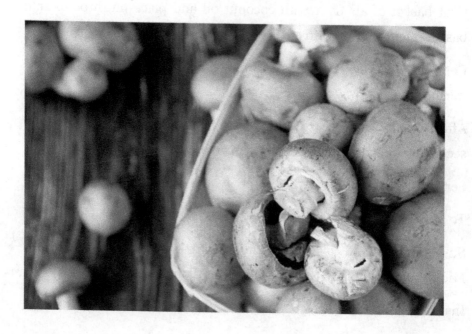

TASTY HOME FRIES

Cooking Time: 20 min   Servings:2

Ingredients

1 tsp. salt

Three russet potatoes, cubed

1 tsp. chili powder

3 tbsp. of paprika seasoning

Olive oil - 2 tbsp.

Pepper - 1/2 tsp.

Garlic powder - 3 tbsp.

Instructions

First to heat, set the temperature of the air fryer to 400°F. Prepare the potatoes by scrubbing and chopping them into cubes.

Then use a glass dish, combine the cubed potatoes with paprika, olive oil, chili powder, and garlic powder until integrated.

In a single layer, assemble the potatoes in the air fryer basket. Fry for approximately 25 minutes.

Then open the lid about every 10 minutes to toss the potatoes for it to be cooked fully.

Remove from the basket and distribute to a serving dish, then serve immediately.

AIR FRYER LEMON ZUCCHINI

ingredients

6-7 cups zucchini (or about 6 small zucchini or 3 large zucchini), sliced into ⅛" thick coins; slice into half-coins if using large zucchini

1 tablespoon olive oil

¼ teaspoon salt

2 lemon slices (or 1.5 teaspoons lemon juice)

instructions

Preheat your air fryer to 400 degrees for 4-5 minutes.

In a medium-size mixing bowl, toss together the zucchini and olive oil until the zucchini is evenly coated in the oil. Sprinkle the salt on and toss the zucchini again until the salt is evenly distributed.

Add the zucchini to the preheated air fryer and air fry for 18-22 minutes, tossing the zucchini every 4 minutes, or until the zucchini is fried to your preferred level of doneness. I like mine super crispy and golden and usually roast for 20-22 minutes.

Squeeze the lemon juice over the zucchini, season the vegetables with extra salt if needed, and serve hot!

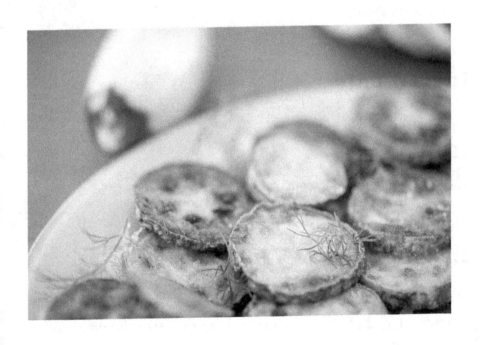

LOW CARB AIR FRYER SAUSAGE BALLS

Prep Time: 18 minutes

 Cook Time: 5 minutes

Total Time: 23 minutes

Servings: 20 Piece

Ingredients

1 pound Ground Pork Sausage

1 cup Almond Flour

1 cup Shredded Cheddar Cheese

Instructions

Prepare Your Air Fryer: Grease your air fryer basket by spraying some avocado oil on the bottom. I also like using a piece of aluminum foil on the bottom in order for the oil to catch which makes for an easy clean up. You can preheat the air fryer, but it is not necessary.

Mix All Ingredients: In a medium sized bowl, add the ground sausage, cheese and almond flour and mix with your hands until all ingredients are evenly combined.

Form Sausage Balls: Form meat mixture into 1-inch balls. You could make them bigger or smaller, however make sure you adjust your

Add each sausage ball in a single layer to the basket of your air fryer and air fry at 375 degrees for 16-18 minutes or until sausage is cooked all the way through.

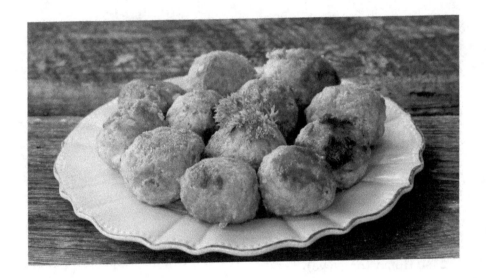

AIR FRYER ROASTED BROCCOLI

Serves: 4

Prep:10 minutes

Cook:20 minutes

TotaL:30 minutes

Ingredients

1 Lb. Broccoli, Cut into florets

1 1/2 Tbsp Peanut oil

1 Tbsp Garlic, minced

Salt

2 Tbsp Reduced sodium soy sauce

2 tsp Honey (or agave)

2 tsp Sriracha

1 tsp Rice vinegar

1/3 Cup Roasted salted peanuts

Fresh lime juice (optional)

Instructions

In a large bowl, toss together the broccoli, peanut oil, garlic and season with sea salt. Make sure the oil covers all the broccoli florets. I like to use my hands to give each one a quick rub.

Spread the broccoli into the wire basket of your air fryer, in as single of a layer, as possible, trying to leave a little bit of space between each floret.

Cook at 400 degrees until golden brown and crispy, about 15 – 20 minutes, stirring halfway.

While the broccoli cooks, mix together the honey, soy sauce, sriracha and rice vinegar in a small, microwave-safe bowl.

Once mixed, microwave the mixture for 10-15 seconds until the honey is melted, and evenly incorporated.

Transfer the cooked broccoli to a bowl and add in the soy sauce mixture. Toss to coat and season to taste with a pinch more salt, if needed.

Stir in the peanuts and squeeze lime on top (if desired.)

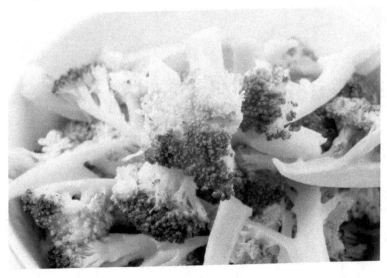

ROASTED BRUSSELS SPROUTS RECIPE

Prep Time: 10 minutes

Cook Time: 8 minutes

Total Time: 18 minutes

Servings: 4 servings

Ingredients

1 lb. brussels sprouts (cleaned and trimmed)

½ tsp. dried thyme

1 tsp. dried parsley

1 tsp. garlic powder (Or 4 cloves, minced)

¼ tsp. salt

2 tsp. oil

Instructions

Place all ingredients in a medium to large mixing bowl and toss to coat the brussels sprouts evenly.

Pour them into the food basket of the air fryer and close it up.

Set the heat to 390 F. and the time to 8 minutes. This setting roasts them nicely on the outside while leaving the insides a nicely cooked al dente.

Cool slightly and serve.

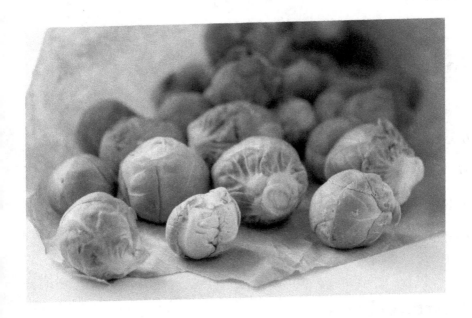

AIR FRYER CHEDDAR JALAPENO POPPERS

Prep time 10 minutes

Cook Time5 minutes

Total Time15 minutes

Servings5

Ingredients

10 fresh jalapenos

6 oz cream cheese I used reduced-fat

1/4 cup shredded cheddar cheese

2 slices bacon cooked and crumbled

cooking oil spray

Instructions

Slice the jalapenos in half, vertically, to create 2 halves per jalapeno.

Place the cream cheese in a bowl. Microwave for 15 seconds to soften.

Remove the seeds and the inside of the jalapeno. (Save some of the seeds if you prefer spicy poppers)

Combine the cream cheese, crumbled bacon, and shredded cheese in a bowl. Mix well.

For extra spicy poppers, add some of the seeds as noted above to the cream cheese mixture, and mix well.

Stuff each of the jalapenos with the cream cheese mixture.

Load the poppers into the Air Fryer. Spray the poppers with cooking oil.

Close the Air Fryer. Cook the poppers on 370 degrees for 5 minutes.

Remove from the Air Fryer and cool before serving.

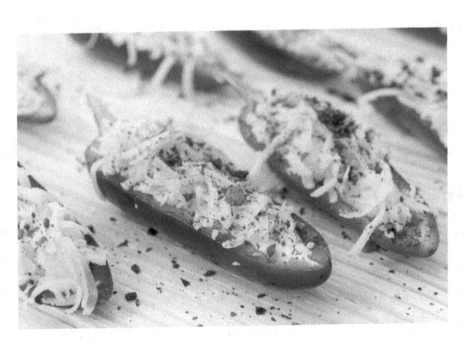

AIR FRYER BANANA BREAD

Total time: 30 minutes

Ingredients

1 el peanut oil or sunflower oil

2 ripe bananas

250 g flower

1 tl baking powder

115 g soft butter

110 g Brown sugar

100 g grated coconut

1 little hand pecans

1 Chilli (finely chopped without seeds)

2 beaten eggs

1 pinch salt

Garnish

1 ripe banana

grater of 1 orange

Instructions

Coat the XXL baking accessory with a little bit of oil.

Put all ingredients in a blender or mix the flour, baking powder and salt in a bowl. Mix the softened butter with the sugar in another bowl.

Mash the bananas with a fork (the riper the bananas, the easier this is) and mix in the beaten eggs. The finer you practice the bananas, the fewer pieces of bananas you will taste in the cake.

Add the banana-egg mixture to the sugar-butter mixture and mix well with a spatula or spoon, also add the chopped chili pepper and the coconut.

Add the flour mixture little by little, mixing again and again, then add the pecans and mix well.

Put the mixture in the XXL baking accessory and place in the Air fryer basket and bake at 160 °C for 30-35 minutes.

Check after 30 minutes if it is done by inserting a skewer; if it comes out clean, it is ready. Otherwise, put an extra 5 minutes in the Air fryer.

When the banana bread has cooled, cut a slice and grate your orange zest over it.

Enjoy!

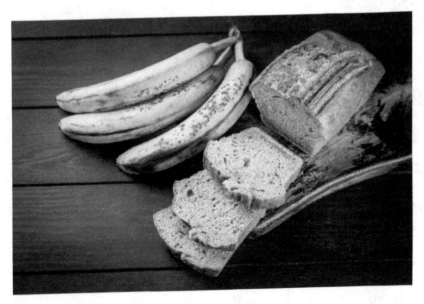

AIR FRYER TEXAS TOAST STICKS

Cooking Time: 5 Min

Servings: 15

Ingredients

- Four pieces of slightly stale thick bread, like Texas toast
- Parchment paper
- Two eggs, lightly crushed
- 1/4 cup milk

(optional)   • 1 tsp. vanilla extract

- 1 tsp. cinnamon
- One pinch of ground nutmeg

Instructions

First slice each piece of bread into thirds to create sticks. Cut a sheet of parchment paper to fit the base of the air fryer basket.

Preheat air fryer to 360 degrees F (180 degrees C).

Mix together eggs, vanilla, vanilla extract, cinnamon, and nutmeg in a bowl till well blended. Into the egg mixture, dip each slice of bread, ensuring every piece is nicely submerged. Shake every breadstick to get rid of excess liquid and set it in one layer in the air fryer basket. Cook in batches, if necessary, to prevent overcrowding the fryer.

Then cook for 5 minutes, then turn bread bits and cook for another five minutes.

BAKED EGG AND HAM CUP

Cooking Time: 10 min

Servings: 2

Ingredients:

•1 egg

•1 cup ham, chopped

•½ onion, chopped

•1 tbsp. butter

•1/3 cup parmesan, grated

Instructions

Start by preheating your fryer to 350°F.

Then whisk the egg into a bowl well before adding in the ham, onion, and butter. Combine well and add seasoning if desired.

Scoop equal portions into three ramekins, adding a sprinkle of parmesan on top.

Then place into the fryer and cook for ten minutes. Take care when removing the ramekins, and serve hot.

AIR FRIED TASTY CHICKEN DRUMSTICKS

Prep time: 5 minutes

Cook time: 25 minutes

Total time: 30 minutes

Ingredients

8 chicken drumsticks

2 tbsp olive oil

1 tsp celtic sea salt

1 tsp fresh cracked pepper

1 tsp garlic powder

1 tsp paprika

1/2 tsp cumin

Instructions

In a small bowl, combine herbs and spices.

Set aside.

Place drumsticks in a bowl or a plastic bag and drizzle with olive oil.

Toss to coat.

Sprinkle herbs and spices all over drumsticks to coat them.

Preheat air fryer at 400 for 2-10 minutes.

Place drumsticks in air fryer basket and cook for 10 minutes on 400.

Remove basket and flip chicken drumsticks.

Cook at 400 for another 10 minutes.

If chicken is not 165 degrees internally, add another 5 minutes of cook-time.

Time can vary based on drumstick size, so do check the temperature with a digital thermometer after cooking to prevent over or under cooking.

When chicken has reached 165 degrees internally, serve immediately.

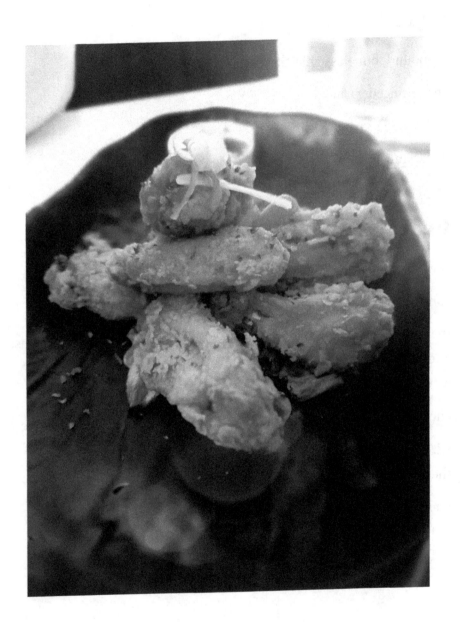

MINCED GARLIC MEATBALLS

Cooking time: 20 min Servings: 4

Ingredients:

½ -pound. boneless chicken thighs

1 tsp. minced garlic

one ¼ cup roasted pecans

½ cup mushrooms

1 tsp. extra virgin olive oil

Instruction

start by preheating your fryer to 375°f.

cube the chicken thighs.

then position them in the food processor along with the garlic, pecans, and other seasonings as desired. pulse until a smooth consistency is achieved.

chop the mushrooms finely. add to the chicken mixture and combine.

with the use of your hands, shape the mixture into balls and brush them with olive oil.

and put the balls into the fryer and cook for eighteen minutes. serve hot.

CRISPY SOUTHERN FRIED CHICKEN

Cooking Time: 25 min

Servings: 6

Ingredients

2 x 6-oz. boneless skinless chicken breasts

2 tbsp. hot sauce

½ tsp. onion powder

1 tbsp. chili powder

2 oz. pork rinds, finely ground

Instruction

Start Slicing the chicken breasts in ½ lengthwise and rub in the hot sauce. Then combine the onion powder with the chili powder, and then rub it into the chicken. Let it marinate for at least a half-hour.

After that use the ground pork rinds to coat the chicken breasts in the ground pork rinds, covering them thoroughly. Place the chicken in your fryer.

Set the fryer at 350°F and cook the chicken for 13 minutes. Turnover the chicken and cook the other side for another 13 minutes or until golden.

Test the chicken with a meat thermometer and when it is fully cooked, it should reach 165°F. Serve hot with the sides of your choice.

ROASTED BRUSSELS SPROUTS

Preparation Time: 8 minutes Cooking Time: 20 minutes Servings: 4

Ingredients:

1 pound fresh Brussels sprouts

1 tbsp. olive oil

½ tsp. salt

1/8 tsp. pepper

¼ cup grated Parmesan cheese

Instructions

Cut the bottoms from the Brussels sprouts and pull off any discolored leaves. Toss with the olive oil, salt, and pepper, and place in the air fryer basket.

Roast for 20 minutes, shaking the air fryer basket twice during the cooking time until the Brussels sprouts are dark golden brown and crisp.

Move the Brussels sprouts to a serving dish and toss with the Parmesan cheese. Serve immediately.

Did You Know? Brussels sprouts were cultivated in Roman times and introduced into the United States in the 1880s. Most Brussels sprouts in this country are grown in California.

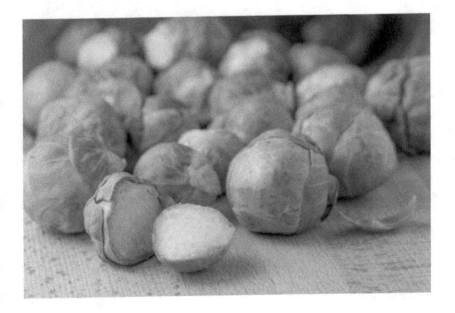

RASPBERRY-EGG FRENCH TOAST

Cooking Time: 8 min

Servings: 4

Ingredients:

- 4 (1-inch-thick) slices French bread
- 2 tbsps. raspberry jam
- 1/3 cup fresh raspberries
- Two egg yolks
- 1/3 cup 2% milk
- 1 tbsp. sugar
- ½ tsp. vanilla extract
- 3 tbsps. sour cream

Instructions

First on either side of each bread slice, cut a pocket, making sure you don't cut through to the other side.

And in a small bowl, combine the raspberry jam and raspberries and crush the raspberries into the jam with a fork.

Then add in a shallow bowl, beat the egg yolks with the milk, sugar, and vanilla until combined.

Spread some of the sour creams in the pocket you cut in the bread slices, and then add the raspberry mixture. Squeeze the edges of the bread slightly to close the opening.

And the dip the bread in the egg mixture, letting the bread stand in the egg for 3 minutes. Flip the bread over and let it stand on the other side for 3 minutes.

Set or preheat the air fryer to 375°F. Arrange the stuffed bread in the air fryer basket in a single layer.

Air fry for 5 minutes, then carefully flip the bread slices and cook for another 3 to 6 minutes, until the French toast is golden brown.

TASTY PEPPER EGG BITES

Cooking Time: 15 min

Servings: 7

Ingredients:

•Five large eggs, beaten

•3 tbsps. 2% milk

•½ tsp. dried marjoram

•1/8 tsp. salt

•Pinch freshly ground black pepper

•1/3 cup minced bell pepper, any color

•3 tbsps. minced scallions

•½ cup shredded Colby or Muenster cheese

Instructions

Then combine the eggs, milk, marjoram, salt, and black pepper in a medium bowl, mix until combined.

Stir in the bell peppers, scallions, and cheese. Fill the seven egg bite cups with the egg mixture, making sure you get some of the solids in each cup. Set or preheat the air fryer to 325°F.

Make a foil sling: Fold an 18-inch-long piece of heavy-duty aluminum foil lengthwise into thirds. Put the egg bite pan on this sling and lower it into the air fryer.

After that leave the foil in the air fryer, but bend down the edges to fit in the appliance.

Bake the egg bites for 10 to 15 minutes or until a toothpick inserted into the center comes out clean.

Use the foil sling to remove the egg bite pan. Let cool for 5 minutes, and then invert the pan onto a plate to remove the egg bites. Serve warm.

SUMMER SQUASH FRITTATA

Cooking Time:25 min

Servings: 4

Ingredients

•¼ cup chopped red bell pepper

•¼ cup chopped yellow summer squash

•2 tbsps. chopped scallion

•2 tbsps. butter

•Five large eggs, beaten

•¼ tsp. sea salt

•1/8 tsp. freshly ground black pepper

•1 cup shredded Cheddar cheese, divided

Instructions

In a 7-inch cake pan, combine the bell pepper, summer squash, and scallion. Add the butter.

Start by preheating the air fryer to 350°F. Set the cake pan in the air fryer basket. Cook the vegetables for 3 to 4 minutes or until they are crisp- tender. Remove the pan from the air fryer.

And use salt and pepper, beat the eggs in a medium bowl. Stir in half of the Cheddar. Pour into the pan with the vegetables.

Then return the pan to the air fryer, cook for 10 to 15 minutes, and then top the frittata with the remaining cheese. Cook for another 4 to 5 minutes or until the cheese is melted and the frittata is set. Cut into wedges to serve.

PAPRIKA CHICKEN LEGS

Prep Time

10 mins

Cook Time

20 mins

Total Time

30 mins

Servings: 4 Calories: 245kcal

Ingredients

6-8 chicken drumsticks

2 tablespoons olive oil

1/2 teaspoon paprika

1/2 teaspoon garlic powder

1/2 teaspoon salt

1/4 teaspoon ground black pepper

Instructions

Preheat air fryer for 2-5 minutes.

Pat drumsticks dry with paper towel. In a small bowl, mix paprika, garlic powder, salt and pepper.

Place chicken in a large bowl or food storage bag. Pour oil and spices over chicken. Mix around until chicken is coated.

Add chicken to air fryer basket. Cook at 390 degrees for 10 minutes. Flip drumsticks over and cook for another 10 minutes at 390 degrees F.

Serve warm.

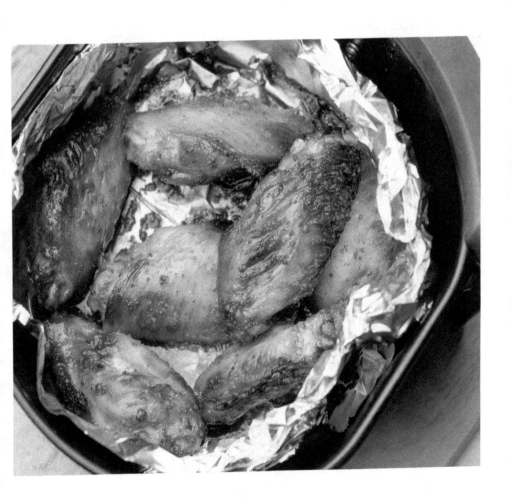

DELICIOUS PAPRIKA VEGETABLES

Cooking Time: 45 min

Servings:2

Ingredients:

Two garlic cloves, chopped

Three russet potatoes

2 oz. onions, chopped

1/4 cup red peppers, chopped

2 tsp. olive oil

1/4 tsp. salt

2 oz. cup green peppers, chopped

1 tsp. paprika seasoning

6 cups cold water

1/8 tsp. pepper

Instructions

First Scrub the potatoes and remove the skins with a knife or vegetable peeler.

Use a cheese grater to shred the potatoes completely with the largest holes available. Transfer the potatoes to a glass dish.

Then empty the cold water into the dish and saturate for approximately 20 minutes.

Empty the potatoes and remove the moisture thoroughly.

Set the temperature of the air to heat at 400°F.

In an additional glass dish, add potatoes, olive oil, salt, garlic powder, paprika powder, and pepper until completely covered.

Place the potatoes in the air fryer basket and steam for 10 minutes.

Open the lid and combine the onion, garlic, and peppers to the basket. Toss ingredients to incorporate.

Then heat for an additional 10 minutes and take out of the basket.

Wait for approximately 5 minutes before serving.

HEALTHY AIR FRYER CHICKEN FAJITAS

Prep Time: 5 minutes Cook Time: 15 minutes Total Time: 20 minutes

Servings: 8

Ingredients

2 chicken breasts boneless and skinless, cut into strips (around 1 pound/450g)

1 red bell pepper sliced into ½ inch slices

yellow bell pepper sliced into ½ inch slices

1 green bell pepper sliced into ½ inch slices

1 red onion sliced into wedges

3 tablespoons fajita seasoning

1 tablespoon vegetable oil

Instructions

Preheat the Air Fryer to 390°F (200°C).

Drizzle oil over the chicken strips, and season with the fajita seasoning. Toss well and make sure that they're evenly coated with the seasoning. Add the veggies, and season well. Make sure that everything is well coated in fajita seasoning.

Put everything in an Air Fryer basket. Air Fry at for 15 minutes, tossing halfway through.

Serve with warmed tortillas, pico de gallo, avocado slices or guacamole.

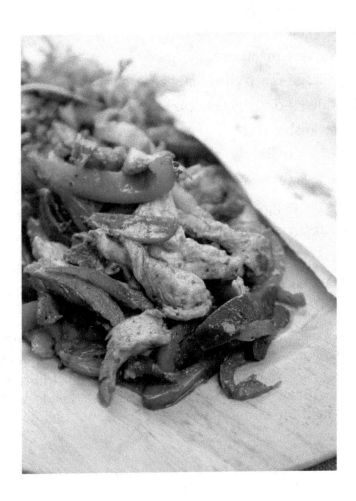

AIR FRYER PASTA WITH CHEESE

Prep Time: 10 minutes

Cook Time: 45 minutes

Ingredients

½ pound dry uncooked pasta (we used elbow macaroni)

2 cups whole milk

1 cup chicken stock

4 tablespoons butter

4 tablespoons cream cheese

8-ounce package sharp cheddar cheese, shredded

1 cup shredded mozzarella cheese

¼ teaspoon kosher salt

¼ teaspoon white pepper

1 teaspoon dry mustard

Pinch Cayenne pepper

Few grinds fresh nutmeg

Instructions

Preheat air fryer on 400 degrees F. for 10 minutes.

Rinse pasta under hot tap water for two minutes and drain.

Place milk, chicken stock, butter and cream cheese in a glass 4-cup or larger measuring cup and microwave until hot, and the butter melted, about 3-4 minutes. (This just needs to be hot enough to melt the butter and cream cheese, not boiling hot)

Mix drained pasta, hot liquid, cheddar, mozzarella, salt, pepper, mustard, cayenne and nutmeg in a large bowl then pour into the Air Fryer handled pan.

Spray a round parchment circle with pan spray and place sprayed side down over the macaroni mixture, pressing down to touch the mixture. Cover the top with foil and set into the heated air fryer and cook for 45 minutes.

Note: Air fryer wattages vary so check at 35 minutes and cook the additional 5-10 minutes as needed. Our air fryer is an 1800-watt air fryer and our macaroni and cheese took exactly 45 minutes.

Remove foil and parchment, stir and serve.

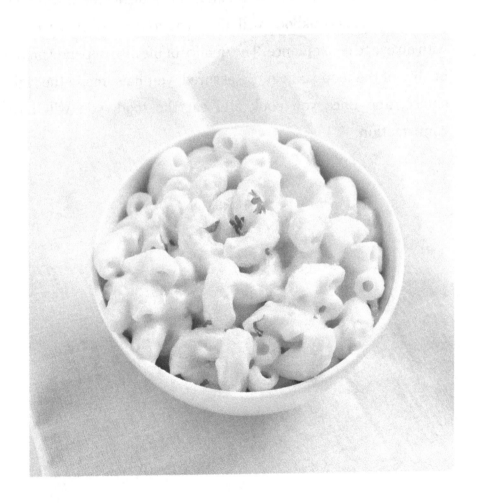

Conclusion

I hope this Air Fryer Cookbook will allow you to understand the features and criteria of this innovative kitchen tool, why you should use it, and how it will change your thinking about food preparation, and a healthier lifestyle. Share these recipes with family and friends, and let them know the advantages of this type of cooking. This cookbook will allow you to get healthy products with an eye to convenience. The quality of life also depends on the quality of the food you eat. Be assured, you have made the right choice, and once you cook and eat the food, you will have confirmation.

*Thank you for
reading this
cookbook*

Violet H. Scott

CPSIA information can be obtained
at www.ICGtesting.com
Printed in the USA
BVHW090117230421
605635BV00001B/159